THE 60-MINUTE

MEDITERRANEAN DIET

COOKBOOK

The Best 50 Mediterranean Recipes for

Diet and Healthy Meal Plans

Healthy & Lovely

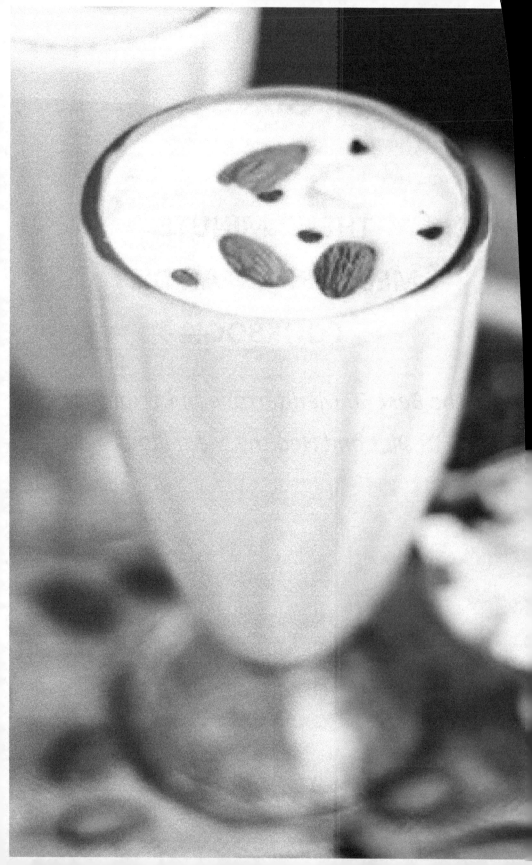

inattention, use, or misuse of the information in question by the reader will render any resulting actions solely under their purview. There are no scenarios in which the publisher or the original author of this work can be in any fashion deemed liable for any hardship or damages that may befall them after undertaking information described herein.

Additionally, the information in the following pages is intended only for informational purposes and should thus be thought of as universal. As befitting its nature, it is presented without assurance regarding its prolonged validity or interim quality. Trademarks that are mentioned are done without written consent and can in no way be considered an endorsement from the trademark holder.

Table of Contents

INTRODUCTION

Mediterranean Diet

A Mediterranean diet incorporates the traditional healthy living habits of people from countries bordering the Mediterranean Sea, including France, Greece, Italy, and Spain. A traditional diet from the Mediterranean region includes a generous portion of fresh produce, whole grains, and legumes, as well as some healthful fats and fish. In general, it's high in vegetables, fruits, legumes, nuts, beans, cereals, grains, fish, and unsaturated fats such as olive oil. It usually includes a low intake of meat and dairy foods.

When you think about Mediterranean food, your mind may go to pizza and pasta from Italy or lamb chops from Greece, but these dishes don't fit into the healthy dietary plans advertised as "Mediterranean." That's how the inhabitants of Crete, Greece, and Southern Italy ate circa 1960, when their rates of chronic disease were among the lowest in the world and their life expectancy among the highest, despite having only limited medical services.

And the real Mediterranean diet is about more than just eating fresh, wholesome food. Daily physical activity and sharing meals with others are vital elements. Together, they can have a profound effect on your mood and mental health and help you foster a deep appreciation for the pleasures of eating healthy and delicious foods.

Of course, making changes to your diet is rarely easy, especially if you're trying to move away from the convenience of processed and takeout foods. But the Mediterranean diet can be an inexpensive as well as a satisfying and very healthy way to eat. Making the switch from pepperoni and pasta to fish and avocados may take some effort, but you could soon be on the path to a healthier and longer life.

If you have a chronic condition like heart disease or high blood pressure, your doctor may even have prescribed it to you. It is often promoted to decrease the risk of heart disease, depression, and dementia.

Research has consistently shown that the Mediterranean diet is effective in reducing the risk of cardiovascular diseases and overall mortality. [3, 4] A study of nearly 26,000 women found that those who followed this type of diet had 25 percent less risk of developing cardiovascular disease over the course of 12 years. [5] The study examined a range of underlying mechanisms that might account for this reduction, and found that changes in inflammation, blood sugar, and body mass index were the biggest drivers.

Tip for Making Your Diet More Mediterranean

You can make your diet more Mediterranean-style by:

- Including fish in your diet
- Choosing products made from vegetable and plant oils, such as olive oil
- Eating plenty of fruit and vegetables
- Eating plenty of starchy foods, such as bread and pasta
- Eating less meat
- Eating less dairy products
- Eating less packaged foods

Avoid the Following Foods If You Are on a Mediterranean Diet

- Foods with added sugars, such as pastries, sodas, and candies
- Refined grains such as white bread, white pasta, and pizza dough containing white flour
- Processed or packaged foods
- Refined oils, which include canola oil and soybean oil
- Deli meats, hot dogs, and other processed meats
- Dairy products

Benefits of Following a Mediterranean Diet

- Can help fight against cancer, diabetes, and cognitive decline
- Reduces the risk of Parkinson's disease
- Increases longevity
- Reduces the risk of Alzheimer's
- Protects against type 2 diabetes
- Prevents heart diseases and strokes
- Keeps you agile

Tips for a Quick Start to a Mediterranean Diet

The easiest way to make the change to a Mediterranean diet is to start with small steps.

You can do this by:

- Limit high-fat dairy by switching to skim or 1% milk.
- Eating more fruits and vegetables by enjoying salad as a starter or side dish, snacking on fruit, and adding veggies to other dishes.
- Choosing whole grains instead of refined breads, rice, and pasta.
- Sautéing food in olive oil instead of butter.
- Substituting fish for red meat at least twice per week.
- Prefer vegetables instead of meat.

1-Week Mediterranean Meal Plan

Monday

Breakfast

Greek yogurt with strawberries and oats

Lunch

Whole-grain sandwich with vegetables

Dinner

A tuna salad, dressed in olive oil, fruit for dessert

Tuesday

Breakfast

Oatmeal with raisins

Lunch

Leftover tuna salad from the night before

Dinner

Salad with tomatoes, olives, and feta cheese

Wednesday

Breakfast

Omelet with veggies, tomatoes and onions, a piece of fruit

Lunch

Whole-grain sandwich with cheese and fresh vegetables

Dinner

Mediterranean lasagna

Thursday

Breakfast

Yogurt with sliced fruits and nuts

Lunch

Leftover lasagna

Dinner

Broiled salmon, served with brown rice and vegetables

Friday

Breakfast

Eggs and vegetables fried in olive oil

Lunch

Greek yogurt with strawberries, oats, and nuts

Dinner

Grilled lamb with salad and baked potato

Saturday

Breakfast

Oatmeal with raisins, nuts, and an apple

Lunch

Whole-grain sandwich with vegetables

Dinner

Mediterranean pizza made with whole wheat, **topped with cheese**, vegetables, and olives

BREAKFAST

Delicious Zucchini Patties with Pancetta

Servings: 6

Preparation Time: 20 minutes

Per Serving: Calories 412, Fat: 29.7g, Total Carbs: 18g, Protein: 27.8g

Ingredients:

- 6 Medium zucchinis, diced
- 12 Slices pancetta
- 12 Eggs
- 2 Tbsps olive oil
- 2 Small onion, chopped
- 2 Tbsps parsley, chopped
- Salt to taste

Procedure:

1. Firstly, cook the pancetta in a skillet over medium heat for 3-5 minutes, until crispy; set aside.
2. Warm the olive oil and cook the onion until soft, for 3 minutes, occasionally stirring.

3. Then, add the zucchinis, and cook for 8 more minutes until zucchini is brown and tender but not mushy.
4. Transfer to a plate and season with salt.
5. Crack the egg into the same skillet and fry over medium heat.
6. Finally, top the zucchini mixture with pancetta slices and a fried egg.
7. Now, serve hot, sprinkled with parsley.

Tempting Carrot Zucchini Bread

Servings: 8

Preparation Time: 70 minutes

Per Serving: Calories 224, Fat 15g; Total Carbs 15g; Protein 11.6g

Ingredients:

- 6 Carrots, shredded
- 1/2 Cup flour
- 2 Tsps vanilla extract
- 12 Eggs
- 2 Tbsps olive oil
- ¾ Tsp baking soda
- 2 Tbsps cinnamon powder
- 1 Tsp salt
- 1 Cup full-fat yogurt
- 2 Tsps apple cider vinegar
- 4 Cups grated zucchini
- 1 Tsp nutmeg powder

Procedure:

1. Firstly, grease the loaf pan with cooking spray. Set aside.
2. Then, mix the carrots, zucchini, flour, vanilla extract, eggs, olive oil, baking soda, cinnamon powder, salt, yogurt, vinegar, and nutmeg.
3. Pour the batter into the loaf pan and bake for 55 minutes at 350ºF.
4. Now, remove the bread after and let cool for 5 minutes.

Butternut Squash Stuffed with Beef and Mushrooms

Servings: 8

Preparation Time: 1 hour

Per Serving: Calories 406, Fat 14.7g; Total Carbs 35.4g; Protein 34g

Ingredients:

- 2 lbs ground beef
- 4 Tbsps olive oil
- 4 lbs butternut squash, pricked with a fork
- Salt and black pepper, to taste
- 6 Garlic cloves, minced
- 4 Green onions, chopped
- 2 Portobello mushrooms, sliced
- 56 Oz canned tomatoes
- ½ Tsp cayenne pepper
- 1 Tsp dried thyme
- 1 lb green beans, halved crosswise

Procedure:

1. First, bake the butternut squash on a lined baking sheet in the oven at 400ºF for 40 minutes.
2. Then, cut in half, set aside to let cool, deseed, scoop out most of the flesh and let sit.
3. Heat olive oil in a pan over medium heat, add in the garlic, mushrooms, green onions, and beef, and cook until the meat browns, about 6-8 minutes.
4. Finally, stir in the green beans, salt, thyme, tomatoes, oregano, black pepper, and cayenne, and cook for 10 minutes; stir in the flesh.
5. Now, stuff the squash halves with the beef mixture, and bake in the oven for 10 minutes

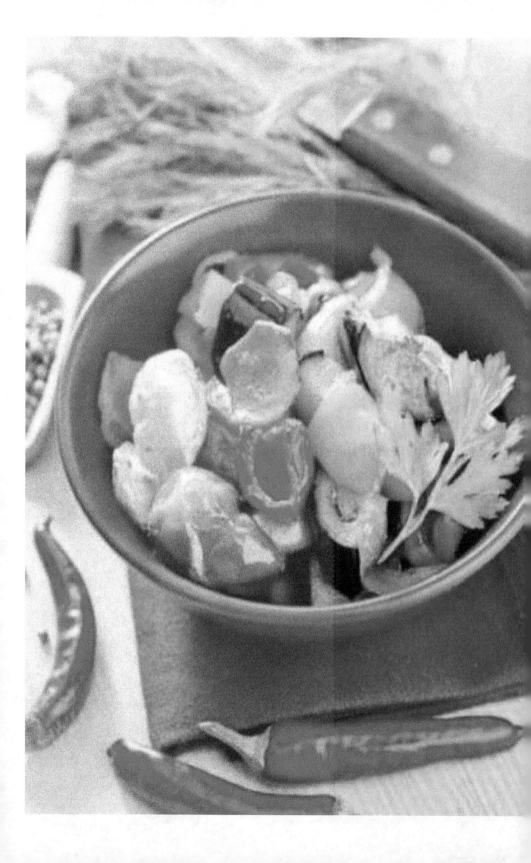

Delectable Vegetable Breakfast Bowl

Servings: 8

Preparation Time: 45 minutes

Per Serving: Calories 213, fat 7.2, fiber 4.8, carbs 34.6, protein 3.6

Ingredients:

- 2 Cups sweet potatoes, peeled, chopped
- 2 Russet potatoes, chopped
- 2 Red onions, sliced
- 4 Bell pepper, trimmed
- 1 Teaspoon garlic powder
- ¾ Teaspoon onion powder
- 2 Tablespoons olive oil
- 2 Tablespoons Sriracha sauce
- 2 Tablespoons coconut milk

Procedure:

1. First, line the baking tray with baking paper.
2. Then, place the chopped russet potato and sweet potato in the tray.

3. Add onion, bell peppers, and sprinkle the vegetables with olive oil, onion powder, and garlic powder.
4. Finally, mix up the vegetables well with the help of the fingertips and transfer in the preheated to the 360F oven.
5. Bake the vegetables for 45 minutes.
6. Meanwhile, make the sauce: mix up together Sriracha sauce and coconut milk.
7. Now, transfer the cooked vegetables in the serving plates and sprinkle them with sriracha sauce.

Delightful Breakfast Green Smoothie

Servings: 4

Preparation Time: 10 minutes

Per Serving: Calories 107, fat 3.6, fiber 2.4, carbs 15.5, protein 4.8

Ingredients:

- 4 Cups spinach
- 4 Cups kale
- 2 Cups bok choy
- 3 Cups organic almond milk
- 2 Tablespoons almonds, chopped
- 1 Cup of water

Procedure:

1. Firstly, place all ingredients in the blender and blend until you get a smooth mixture.
2. Then, pour the smoothie in the serving glasses.
3. Now, add ice cubes if desired.

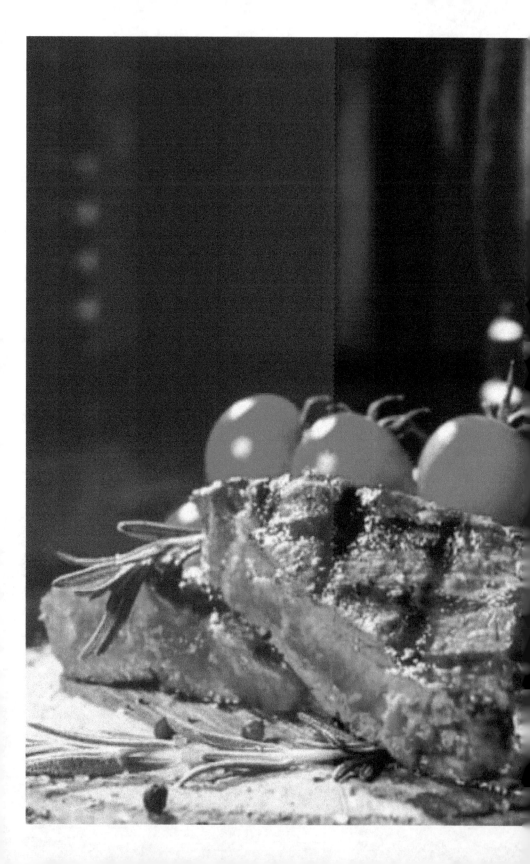

Steak

Servings: 4

Preparation Time: 25 minutes

Per Serving: Calories 301, Total Fat 25.1, Total Carbs 0, Protein 19.1g, Sugar 0g, Sodium 65mg

Ingredients:

- 1 lb steak, quality - cut
- Salt and freshly cracked black pepper

Procedure:

1. First, switch on the air fryer, set frying basket in it, then set its temperature to 385°F and let preheat.
2. Then, meanwhile, prepare the steaks, and for this, season steaks with salt and freshly cracked black pepper on both sides.
3. When air fryer has preheated, add prepared steaks in the fryer basket, shut it with a lid and cook for 15 minutes.
4. When done, transfer steaks to a dish and then serve immediately.

5. For meal prepping, evenly divide the steaks between two heatproof containers, close them with a lid and refrigerate for up to 3 days until ready to serve.
6. Now, when ready to eat, reheat steaks into the microwave until hot and then serve.

Almond Crusted Rack Lamb with Rosemary

Servings: 4

Preparation Time: 45 minutes

Per Serving: Calories 471, Total Fat 31.6g, Total Carbs 8.5g, Protein 39g, Sugar 1.5g, Sodium 145mg

Ingredients:

- 2 Garlic cloves, minced
- 1 tbsp olive oil
- Salt and freshly cracked black pepper
- ¾ lb rack of lamb
- 2 Small organic eggs
- 2 Tbsps breadcrumbs
- 4 Oz almonds, finely chopped
- 1 tbsp fresh rosemary, chopped

Procedure:

1. First, switch on the oven and set its temperature to 350°F, and let it preheat.
2. Then, meanwhile, take a baking tray, grease it with oil, and set it aside until required.

3. Mix garlic, oil, salt, and freshly cracked black pepper in a bowl and coat the rack of lamb with this garlic, rub on all sides.

4. Crack the egg in a bowl, whisk until blended, and set aside until required.

5. Place breadcrumbs in another dish, add almonds and rosemary and stir until mixed.

6. Dip the seasoned rack of lamb with egg, dredge with the almond mixture until evenly coated on all sides and then place it onto the prepared baking tray.

7. When the oven has preheated, place the rack of lamb in it, and cook for 35 minutes until thoroughly cooked.

8. When done, take out the baking tray, transfer the rack of lamb onto a dish, and serve straight away.

9. For meal prep, cut rack of lamb into pieces, evenly divide the lamb between two heatproof containers, close them with lid and refrigerate for up to 3 days until ready to serve.

10. Finally, when ready to eat, reheat the rack of lamb in the microwave until hot and then serve.

Tasty Cheesy Eggs in Avocado

Servings: 4

Preparation Time: 35 minutes

Per Serving: Calories 210, Total Fat 16.6g, Total Carbs 6.4g, Protein 10.7g, Sugar 2.2g, Sodium 151mg

Ingredients:

- 2 Medium avocadoes
- 4 Organic eggs
- 1/2 Cup shredded cheddar cheese
- Salt and freshly cracked black pepper
- 2 Tbsps olive oil

Procedure:

1. Firstly, switch on the oven, then set its temperature to 425°F, and let preheat.
2. Meanwhile, prepare the avocados and for this, cut the avocado in half and remove its pit.
3. Then, take two muffin tins, grease them with oil, and then add an avocado half into each tin.

4. Crack an egg into each avocado half, season well with salt and freshly cracked black pepper, and then sprinkle cheese on top.

5. When the oven has preheated, place the muffin tins in the oven and bake for 15 minutes until cooked.

6. Now, when done, take out the muffin tins, transfer the avocados baked organic eggs to a dish, and then serve them.

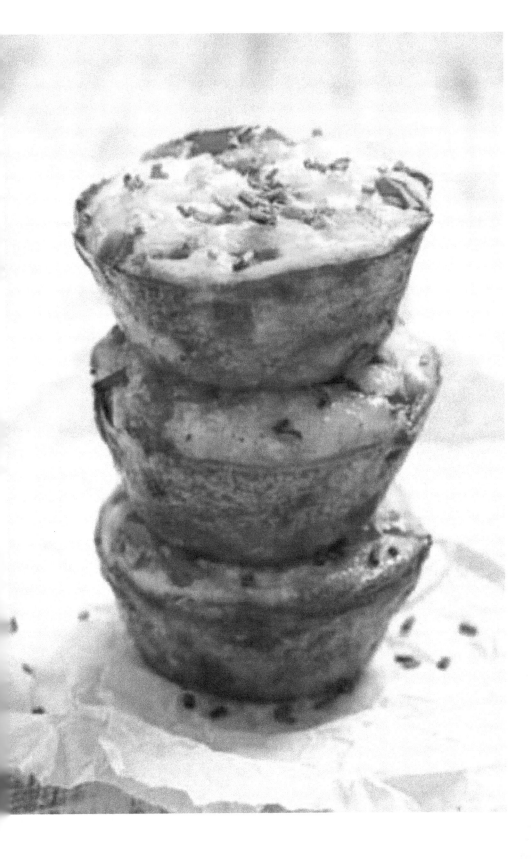

Delicious Leeks Eggs Muffins

Servings: 4

Preparation Time: 20 minutes

Per Serving: calories 308, fat 19.4, fiber 1.7, carbs 8.7, protein 24.4

Ingredients:

- 6 Eggs, whisked
- 1/2 Cup baby spinach
- 4 Tablespoons leeks, chopped
- 8 Tablespoons parmesan, grated
- 4 Tablespoons almond milk
- Cooking spray
- 2 Small red bell peppers, chopped
- Salt and black pepper to the taste
- 2 Tomatoes, cubed
- 4 tablespoons cheddar cheese, grated

Procedure:

1. Firstly, in a bowl, combine the eggs with the milk, salt, pepper and the rest of the ingredients except the cooking spray and whisk well.
2. Then, grease a muffin tin with the cooking spray and divide the eggs mixture in each muffin mould.
3. Now, bake at 380 degrees F for 20 minutes and serve them for breakfast.

Tempting Mango and Spinach Bowls

Servings: 8

Preparation Time: 10 minutes

Per Serving: calories 211, fat 4.5, fiber 6.5, carbs 10.2, protein 3.5

Ingredients:

- 2 Cups baby arugula
- 2 Cups baby spinach, chopped
- 2 Mangoes, peeled and cubed
- 2 Cups strawberries, halved
- 2 Tablespoons hemp seeds
- 2 Cucumbers, sliced
- 2 Tablespoons lime juice
- 2 Tablespoons tahini paste
- 2 Tablespoons water

Procedure:

1. Firstly, in a salad bowl, mix the arugula with the rest of the ingredients except the tahini and the water and toss.

2. Then, in a small bowl, combine the tahini with the water, whisk well, add to the salad, toss, divide into small bowls and serve for breakfast.

Delicious Veggie Quiche

Servings: 4

Preparation Time: 55 minutes

Per Serving: calories 211, fat 14.4, fiber 1.4, carbs 12.5, protein 8.6

Ingredients:

- 1 Cup sun-dried tomatoes, chopped
- 2 Prepared pie crust
- 4 Tablespoons avocado oil
- 2 Yellow onions, chopped
- 4 Garlic cloves, minced
- 4 Cups spinach, chopped
- 2 Red bell peppers, chopped
- 1 Cup kalamata olives, pitted and sliced
- 2 Teaspoons parsley flakes
- 2 Teaspoosn oregano, dried
- 1 Cup feta cheese, crumbled
- 8 Eggs, whisked
- 3 Cups almond milk
- 2 Cups cheddar cheese, shredded

- Salt and black pepper to the taste

Procedure:

1. Firstly, heat up a pan with the oil over medium-high heat, add the garlic and onion and sauté for 3 minutes.
2. Then, add the bell pepper and sauté for 3 minutes more.
3. Add the olives, parsley, spinach, oregano, salt and pepper and cook everything for 5 minutes.
4. Finally, add tomatoes and the cheese, toss and take off the heat.
5. Arrange the pie crust in a pie plate, pour the spinach and tomatoes mix inside and spread.
6. In a bowl, mix the eggs with salt, pepper, milk and half of the cheese, whisk and pour over the mixture in the pie crust.
7. Sprinkle the remaining cheese on top and bake at 375 degrees F for 40 minutes.
8. Now, cool the quiche down, slice and serve for breakfast.

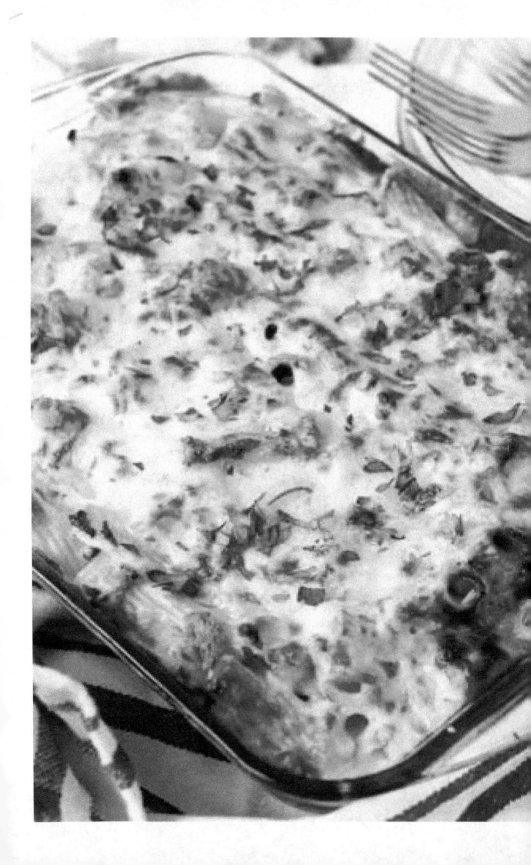

Yummy Tuna and Cheese Bake

Servings: 8

Preparation Time: 15 minutes

Per Serving: calories 283, fat 14.2, fiber 5.6, carbs 12.1, protein 6.4

Ingredients:

- 20 Ounces canned tuna, drained and flaked
- 8 Eggs, whisked
- 1 Cup feta cheese, shredded
- 2 Tablespoons chives, chopped
- 2 Tablespoons parsley, chopped
- Salt and black pepper to the taste
- 6 Teaspoons olive oil

Procedure:

1. Firstly, grease a baking dish with the oil, add the tuna and the rest of the ingredients except the cheese, toss and bake at 370 degrees F for 15 minutes.
2. Then, sprinkle the cheese on top, leave the mix aside for 5 minutes, slice and serve for breakfast.

Enticing Blackberry Yogurt Green Smoothie

Servings: 4

Preparation Time: 5 minutes

Per Serving: calories: 201 | fat: 14.5g | protein: 7.1g | carbs: 14.9g | fiber: 4.3g | sodium: 103mg

Ingredients:

- 2 Cups plain Greek yogurt
- 2 Cups baby spinach
- 1 Cup frozen blackberries
- 1 Cup unsweetened almond milk
- 1 Teaspoon peeled and grated fresh ginger
- 1/2 Cup chopped pecans

Procedure:

1. Firstly, process the yogurt, baby spinach, blackberries, almond milk, and ginger in a food processor until smoothly blended.
2. Then, divide the mixture into two bowls and serve topped with the chopped pecans.

SNACKS

Easy Healthy Kidney Bean Dip

Servings: 12

Preparation Time: 20 minutes

Per Serving: Calories 136 Fat 3.2 g Carbohydrates 20 g Sugar 2.1 g Protein 7.7 g Cholesterol 0 mg

Ingredients:

- 2 Cups dry white kidney beans, soaked overnight and drained
- 2 Tbsps fresh lemon juice
- 4 tbsps water
- 1 Cup coconut yogurt
- 2 Roasted garlic cloves
- 2 Tbsps olive oil
- 1/2 Tsp cayenne
- 2 Tsps dried parsley
- Pepper
- Salt

Procedure:

1. Firstly, add soaked beans and 1 3/4 cups of water into the instant pot.
2. Then, seal the pot with a lid and cook on high for 10 minutes.
3. Once done, allow to release pressure naturally. Remove lid.
4. Drain beans well and transfer them into the food processor.
5. Finally, add the remaining ingredients into the food processor and process until smooth.
6. Now, serve and enjoy.

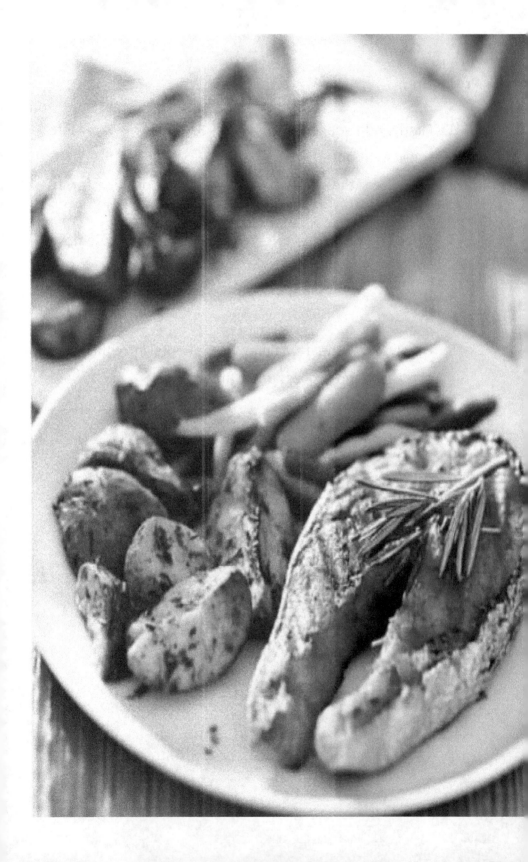

Delectable Salmon with Potatoes

Servings: 8

Preparation Time: 25 minutes

Per Serving: Calories 362 Fat 18.1 g Carbohydrates 14.5 g Sugar 0 g Protein 37.3 g Cholesterol 76 mg

Ingredients:

- 3 lbs Salmon fillets, boneless and cubed
- 4 Tbsps olive oil
- 2 Cups fish stock
- 4 Tbsps parsley, chopped
- 2 Tsps garlic, minced
- 2 lbs baby potatoes, halved
- Pepper
- Salt

Procedure:

1. Firstly, add oil into the inner pot of instant pot and set the pot on sauté mode.
2. Then, add garlic and sauté for 2 minutes.
3. Add remaining ingredients and stir well.

4. Seal pot with lid and cook on high for 13 minutes.
5. Finally, once done, release pressure using quick release. Remove lid.
6. Now, serve and enjoy.

Tasty Ricotta Filled Piquillos

Servings: 8

Preparation Time: 20 minutes

Per Serving:

Ingredients:

- 2 Tbsps olive oil
- 16 Canned roasted piquillo peppers
- 6 Slices Jamon serrano
- 2 Tbsps balsamic vinegar

Filling:

- 16 Oz ricotta cheese
- 2 Eggs, beaten
- 6 Tbsps parsley, chopped
- 2 Garlic clove, minced
- 2 Tbsps olive oil
- 2 Tbsps mint, chopped

Procedure:

1. Firstly, combine all filling ingredients in a bowl. Place in a freezer bag, press down and squeeze, and cut off the bottom. Drain and deseed the peppers.
2. Then, squeeze about 2 tbsps of the filling into each pepper.
3. Wrap a jamon serrano slice onto each pepper.
4. Finally, secure with toothpicks. Arrange them on a serving platter.
5. Now, sprinkle the olive oil and vinegar over.

Pleasant Crispy Zucchini Sticks

Servings: 8

Preparation Time: 20 minutes

Per Serving:

Ingredients:

- 2 Tsps smoked paprika
- 1/2 Cup breadcrumbs
- 1/2 Cup Pecorino Romano cheese, shredded
- Salt and chili pepper to taste
- 6 Fresh eggs
- 8 zucchinis, cut into strips
- Aioli:
- 1 Cup mayonnaise
- 2 Garlic clove, minced
- Juice and zest from ½ lemon

Procedure:

1. Firstly, line a baking sheet with foil. Grease with cooking spray and set aside.

2. Then, mix the breadcrumbs, smoked paprika, Pecorino Romano cheese, salt, and chili pepper in a bowl. Beat the eggs in another bowl. Coat zucchini strips in egg, then in cheese mixture, and arrange on the baking sheet.

3. Grease lightly with cooking spray and bake in the oven for 15 minutes at 425ºF to be crispy.

4. Combine in a bowl mayonnaise, lemon juice, and garlic, and gently stir until everything is well incorporated. Add the lemon zest, adjust the seasoning and stir again.

5. Finally, cover and place in the refrigerator until ready to serve.

6. Now, serve the zucchini strips with garlic aioli for dipping.

Easy Homemade Biscuits with Mascarpone

Servings: 12

Preparation Time: 25 minutes

Per Serving:

Ingredients:

- 14 Tbsps hazelnut liquor
- 12 Egg whites
- 2 Egg yolks, beaten
- 2 Tsps vanilla bean paste
- 16 Oz swerve confectioner's sugar
- 1/2 Tsp salt
- 1/2 Cup fragrant hazelnuts, ground
- Juice of 1 lemon
- 1/2 Cup mascarpone cheese
- 1/2 Cup butter, room temperature
- ¾ Cup confectioner's sugar for topping

Procedure:

1. Firstly, line a baking sheet with parchment paper.

2. In a bowl, beat eggs whites, salt, and vanilla paste while you gradually spoon in 8 oz of swerve confectioner's sugar until a stiff mixture.

3. Add hazelnuts and fold in the egg yolk, lemon juice, and hazelnut liquor.

4. Spoon the mixture into the piping bag and press out 40 to 50 mounds on the baking sheet.

5. Bake the biscuits in the oven for 15 minutes at 300ºF by which time they should be golden brown.

6. Whisk the mascarpone cheese, butter, and swerve confectioner's sugar set aside.

7. When the biscuits are ready, transfer them into a serving bowl and let cool.

8. Finally, spread a scoop of mascarpone cream onto one biscuit and snap with another biscuit.

9. Now, sift some confectioner's sugar on top of them and serve.

Flavorful Chicken Fritters with Rosemary Dip

Servings: 8

Preparation Time: 40 minutes

Per Serving:

Ingredients:

- 8 Tbsps rosemary, chopped
- 4 Chicken breasts, thinly sliced
- 3 Cups mayonnaise
- 1/2 Cup flour
- 4 Eggs
- Salt and black pepper to taste
- 2 Cups mozzarella cheese, grated
- 6 Tbsps olive oil
- 2 Cups buttermilk
- 2 Tsps garlic powder
- 2 Tbsps parsley, chopped
- 1 Onion, chopped

Procedure:

1. Firstly, mix the chicken, ¼ cup of mayonnaise, flour, eggs, salt, pepper, mozzarella, and 1 tbsp of rosemary, in a bowl.
2. Then, cover the bowl with plastic wrap and refrigerate it for 2 hours.
3. After the marinating time is over, remove it from the fridge.
4. In a bowl, mix the remaining mayonnaise, remaining rosemary, buttermilk, garlic powder, onion, and salt.
5. Cover the bowl with plastic wrap and refrigerate for 30 minutes.
6. Place a skillet over medium fire and heat the olive oil.
7. Fetch 2 tablespoons of chicken mixture into the skillet, use the back of a spatula to flatten the top. Cook for 4 minutes, flip, and fry for 4 more.
8. Finally, remove onto a wire rack and repeat the cooking process until the batter is finished, adding more oil as needed.
9. Now, garnish the fritters with parsley and serve with rosemary dip.

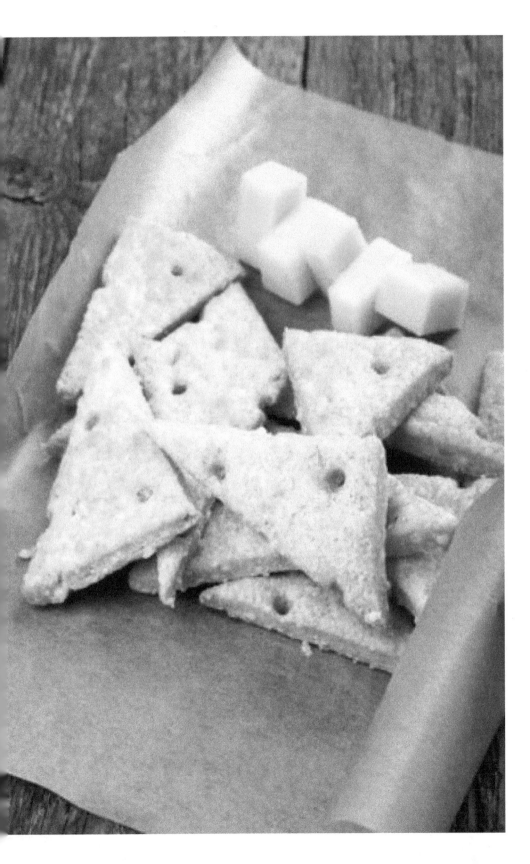

Tempting Cheesy Cracker

Servings: 12

Preparation Time: 25 minutes

Per Serving:

Ingredients:

- 3 Cups flour
- 20 Oz Spanish Manchego cheese, grated
- Salt and black pepper to taste
- 2 Tsps garlic powder
- 8 Tbsps olive oil
- 1/2 Tsp sweet paprika
- ⅓ Cup heavy cream

Procedure:

1. Firstly, mix the flour, manchego cheese, salt, pepper, garlic powder, and paprika in a bowl. Add in the olive oil and mix well.
2. Then, top with the heavy cream and mix again until a smooth, thick mixture has formed.
3. Add 1 to 2 tablespoons of water if it is too thick.

4. Place the dough on a cutting board and cover it with plastic wrap. Use a rolling pin to spread out the dough into a light rectangle.
5. Finally, cut cracker squares out of the dough and arrange them on a baking sheet without overlapping.
6. Now, bake in the oven for 20 minutes at 350ºF; serve chilled.

Pleasant Rosemary Cauliflower Dip

Servings: 8

Preparation Time: 25 minutes

Per Serving: Calories 128 Fat 9.4 g Carbohydrates 10.4 g Sugar 4 g Protein 3.1 g Cholesterol 21 mg

Ingredients:

- 2 lb cauliflower florets
- 2 Tbsps fresh parsley, chopped
- 1 Cup heavy cream
- 1 Cup vegetable stock
- 2 Tbsps garlic, minced
- 2 Tbsps rosemary, chopped
- 2 Tbsps olive oil
- 2 Onions, chopped
- Pepper
- Salt

Procedure:

1. Firstly, add oil into the inner pot of instant pot and set the pot on sauté mode.

2. Then, add onion and sauté for 5 minutes.
3. Add remaining ingredients except for parsley and heavy cream and stir well.
4. Seal pot with lid and cook on high for 10 minutes.
5. Once done, allow to release pressure naturally for 10 minutes, then release remaining using quick release. Remove lid.
6. Finally, add cream and stir well. Blend cauliflower mixture using immersion blender until smooth.
7. Now, garnish with parsley and serve.

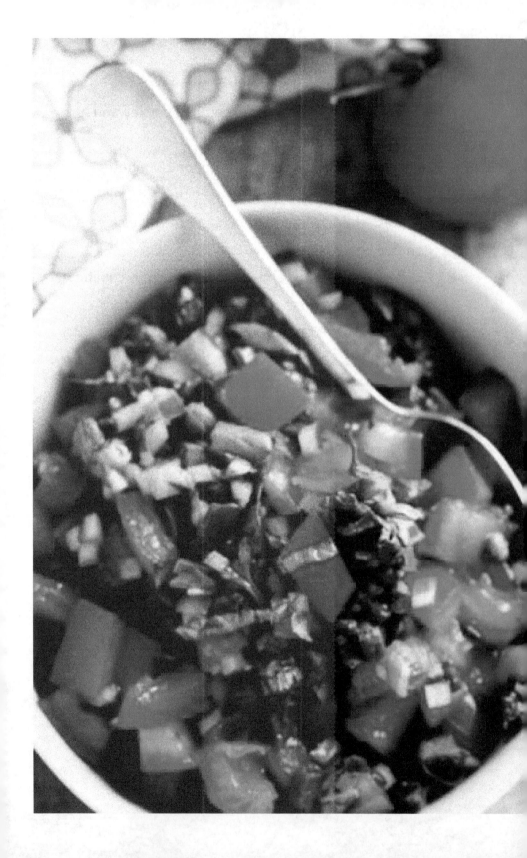

Tempting Tomato Olive Salsa

Servings: 8

Preparation Time: 15 minutes

Per Serving: Calories 119 Fat 10.8 g Carbohydrates 6.5 g Sugar 1.3 g Protein 1.2 g Cholesterol 0 mg

Ingredients:

- 4 Cups olives, pitted and chopped
- 1/2 Cup fresh parsley, chopped
- 1/2 Cup fresh basil, chopped
- 4 Tbsps green onion, chopped
- 2 Cups grape tomatoes, halved
- 2 Tbsps olive oil
- 2 Tbsps vinegar
- Pepper
- Salt

Procedure:

1. Firstly, add all ingredients into the inner pot of instant pot and stir well.
2. Seal pot with lid and cook on high for 5 minutes.

3. Then, once done, allow to release pressure naturally for 5 minutes, then release remaining using quick release. Remove lid.

4. Now, stir well and serve.

Tasty Balsamic Bell Pepper Salsa

Servings: 2

Preparation Time: 15 minutes

Per Serving: : Calories 235 Fat 14.2 g Carbohydrates 19.8 g Sugar 10.7 g Protein 9.2 g Cholesterol 25 mg

Ingredients:

- 4 Red bell peppers, chopped and seeds removed
- 2 Cups grape tomatoes, halved
- 1 tbsp cayenne
- 2 Tbsps balsamic vinegar
- 4 Cups vegetable broth
- 1 Cup sour cream
- 1 Tsp garlic powder
- 1 Onion, chopped
- Salt

Procedure:

1. First, add all ingredients except cream into the instant pot and stir well.

2. Then, seal the pot with a lid and cook on high for 6 minutes.
3. Once done, release pressure using quick release. Remove lid.
4. Add sour cream and stir well.
5. Finally, blend the salsa mixture using an immersion blender until smooth.

Easy Falafel Balls with Tahini Sauce

Servings: 8

Preparation Time: 2 hours

Per Serving: calories: 574 | fat: 27.1g | protein: 19.8g | carbs: 69.7g | fiber: 13.4g | sodium: 1246mg

Ingredients:

- 1 Cup tahini
- 4 Tablespoons lemon juice
- 1/2 Cup finely chopped flat-leaf parsley
- 4 Cloves garlic, minced
- 1 Cup cold water, as needed
- Falafel:
- 2 Cups dried chickpeas, soaked overnight, drained
- 1/2 Cup chopped flat-leaf parsley
- 1/2 Cup chopped cilantro
- 2 Large onion, chopped
- 1 Teaspoon cumin
- 1 Teaspoon chili flakes
- 8 Cloves garlic
- 2 Teaspoons sea salt

- 10 Tablespoons almond flour
- 3 Teaspoons baking soda, dissolved in 1 teaspoon water
- 4 Cups peanut oil
- 2 Medium bell peppers, chopped
- 2 Medium tomatoes, chopped
- 8 Whole-wheat pita breads

Procedure:

1. Firstly, make the Tahini Sauce
2. Then, combine the ingredients for the tahini sauce in a small bowl.
3. Stir to mix well until smooth.
4. Wrap the bowl in plastic and refrigerate until ready to serve.
5. Make the Falafel
6. Put the chickpeas, parsley, cilantro, onion, cumin, chili flakes, garlic, and salt in a food processor.
7. Pulse to mix well but not puréed.
8. Add the flour and baking soda to the food processor, then pulse to form a smooth and tight dough.
9. Put the dough in a large bowl and wrap in plastic. Refrigerate for at least 2 hours to let it rise.
10. Divide and shape the dough into walnut-sized small balls.

11. Pour the peanut oil in a large pot and heat over high heat until the temperature of the oil reaches 375ºF (190ºC).
12. Drop 6 balls into the oil each time, and fry for 5 minutes or until golden brown and crispy.
13. Turn the balls with a strainer to make them fried evenly.
14. Transfer the balls on paper towels with the strainer, then drain the oil from the balls.
15. Finally, roast the pita breads in the oven for 5 minutes or until golden brown, if needed, then stuff the pitas with falafel balls and top with bell peppers and tomatoes.
16. Now, drizzle with tahini sauce and serve immediately.

Yummy Glazed Mushrooms and Vegetable Fajitas

Servings: 12

Preparation Time: 40 minutes

Per Serving:

Ingredients:

- Spicy Glazed Mushrooms:
- 2 Teaspoons olive oil
- 2 (10- to 12-ounce / 284- to 340-g) package cremini mushrooms, rinsed and drained, cut into thin slices
- 2 Teaspoons chili powder
- Sea salt and freshly ground black pepper, to taste
- 1 Teaspoon maple syrup
- Fajitas:
- 4 Teaspoons olive oil
- 2 onions, chopped
- Sea salt, to taste
- 2 Bell pepper, any color, deseeded and sliced into long strips
- 2 Zucchinis, cut into large matchsticks

- 12 Whole-grain tortilla
- 4 Carrots, grated
- 8 Scallions, sliced
- 1 Cup fresh cilantro, finely chopped

Procedure:

1. Firstly, make the Spicy Glazed Mushrooms
2. Heat the olive oil in a nonstick skillet over medium heat until shimmering.
3. Then, add the mushrooms and sauté for 10 minutes or until tender.
4. Sprinkle the mushrooms with chili powder, salt, and ground black pepper. Drizzle with maple syrup.
5. Stir to mix well and cook for 5 to 7 minutes or until the mushrooms are glazed.
6. Set aside until ready to use.
7. Make the Fajitas
8. Heat the olive oil in the same skillet over medium heat until shimmering.
9. Add the onion and sauté for 5 minutes or until translucent. Sprinkle with salt.
10. Add the bell pepper and zucchini and sauté for 7 minutes or until tender.

11. Meanwhile, toast the tortilla in the oven for 5 minutes or until golden brown.
12. Finally, allow the tortilla to cool for a few minutes until they can be handled, then assemble the tortilla with glazed mushrooms, sautéed vegetables and remaining vegetables to make the fajitas.
13. Now, serve immediately.

Delicious Mini Pork and Cucumber Lettuce Wraps

Servings: 6

Preparation Time: 20 minutes

Per Serving: calories: 78 | fat: 5.6g | protein: 5.5g | carbs: 1.4g | fiber: 0.3g | sodium: 50mg

Ingredients:

- 4 Ounces (227 g) cooked ground pork
- 1/2 Cucumber, diced
- 1/2 Tomato, diced
- 1/2 Red onion, sliced
- 1/2 Ounce (28 g) low-fat feta cheese, crumbled
- Juice of 1 lemon
- 1/2 Tablespoon extra-virgin olive oil
- Sea salt and freshly ground pepper, to taste
- 6 Small, intact iceberg lettuce leaves

Procedure:

1. Firstly, combine the ground pork, cucumber, tomato, and onion in a large bowl, then scatter with feta cheese.
2. Then, drizzle with lemon juice and olive oil, and sprinkle with salt and pepper. Toss to mix well.
3. Finally, unfold the small lettuce leaves on a large plate or several small plates, then divide and top with the pork mixture. Wrap & Serve.

LUNCH

Delicious Baked Italian Sausage with Cheese Topping

Servings: 10

Preparation Time: 25 minutes

Per Serving:

Ingredients:

- 6 Tbsps olive oil
- 32 Oz Italian pork sausage, chopped
- 16 Oz mozzarella cheese, grated
- 2 Onions, sliced
- 8 Sun-dried tomatoes, sliced thin
- Salt and black pepper to taste
- 6 Green bell peppers, seeded and chopped
- 4 Orange bell peppers, seeded and chopped
- A pinch of red pepper flakes
- 4 Tbsps fresh parsley, chopped

Procedure:

1. Firstly, preheat oven to 340ºF.

2. Warm olive oil in a pan over medium heat and cook the sausage slices, for 3 minutes on each side, remove to a bowl, and set aside.
3. Then, stir in the tomatoes, bell peppers, and onion, and cook for 5 minutes.
4. Season with pepper, pepper flakes, and salt and mix well. Cook for 1 minute, and remove from heat.
5. Finally, lay the sausage slices into a baking dish, place the bell peppers mixture on top, scatter with the mozzarella cheese and bake for 10 minutes until the cheese melts.
6. Now, serve topped with parsley.

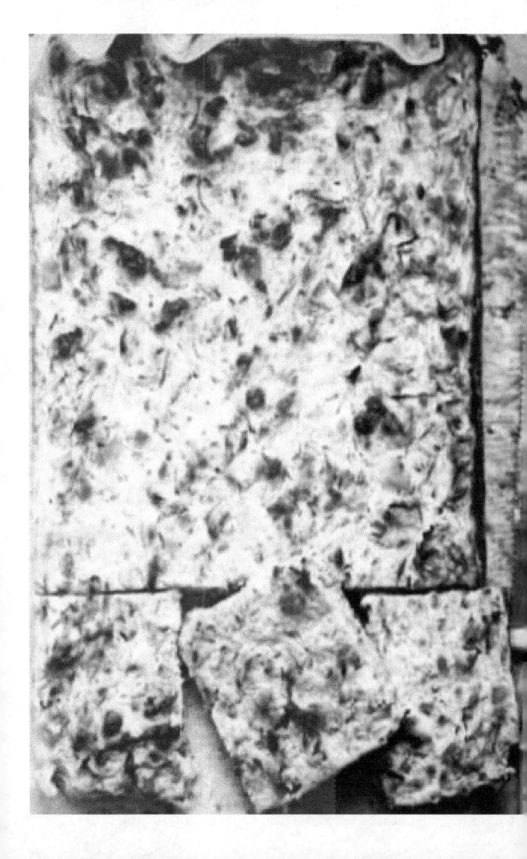

Tempting Vegetable Frittata

Servings: 8

Preparation Time: 25 minutes

Per Serving: Calories 310; Fat: 26.2g; Total Carbs: 13.9g; Protein: 15.4g

Ingredients:

- 4 Tbsps olive oil
- 1 Cup green onions, chopped
- 4 Garlic cloves, minced
- 2 Jalapeño peppers, chopped
- 2 Carrots, chopped
- 2 Zucchinis, chopped
- 2 Bell pepper, seeded and chopped
- 16 Eggs
- Salt and black pepper to taste
- 1 Tsp dried thyme

Procedure:

1. Firstly, preheat the oven to 350ºF.
2. Warm olive oil in a pan over medium heat.

3. Then, stir in green onions and garlic, and sauté for 3 minutes until tender.
4. Pour in carrot, zucchini, bell pepper, and jalapeño pepper, and cook for 4 minutes.
5. Finally, remove the mixture to a greased baking pan with cooking spray.
6. Now, in a bowl, whisk the eggs, season with salt and pepper, and pour over vegetables.
7. Bake for about 18 minutes.

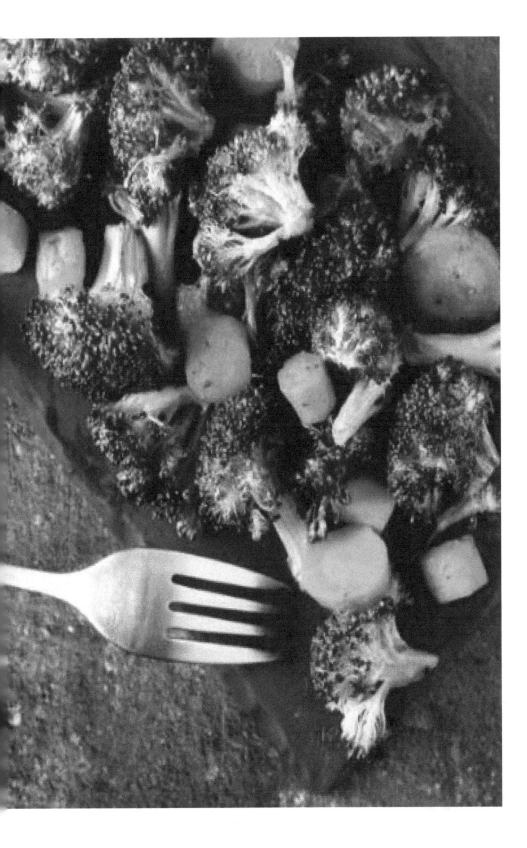

Delectable Vegan Carrots and Broccoli

Servings: 12

Preparation Time: 15 minutes

Per Serving: Calories 51 Fat 2.6 g Carbohydrates 6.3 g Sugar 2.2 g Protein 2 g Cholesterol 0 mg

Ingredients:

- 8 Cups broccoli florets
- 4 Carrots, peeled and sliced
- 1/2 Cup water
- 1 Lemon juice
- 2 Tsps garlic, minced
- 2 Tbsps olive oil
- 1/2 Cup vegetable stock
- 1/2 Tsp Italian seasoning
- Salt

Procedure:

1. Firstly, add oil into the inner pot of instant pot and set the pot on sauté mode.
2. Then, add garlic and sauté for 30 seconds.

3. Add carrots and broccoli and cook for 2 minutes.

4. Add remaining ingredients and stir everything well.

5. Seal pot with lid and cook on high for 3 minutes.

6. Finally, once done, release pressure using quick release.

7. Remove li, stir and serve.

Delightful Zucchini Tomato Potato Ratatouille

Servings: 12

Preparation Time: 20 minutes

Per Serving: Calories 175 Fat 1.9 g

Ingredients:

- 3 lbs potatoes, cut into cubes
- 1 Cup fresh basil
- 56 Oz fire-roasted tomatoes, chopped
- 2 Onions, chopped
- 8 Mushrooms, sliced
- 2 Bell peppers, diced
- 24 Oz eggplant, diced
- 16 Oz zucchini, diced
- 16 Oz yellow squash, diced
- Pepper
- Salt

Procedure:

1. Firstly, add all ingredients except basil into the instant pot and stir well.

2. Then, seal the pot with a lid and cook on high for 10 minutes.
3. Once done, release pressure using quick release.
4. Remove lid.
5. Now, add basil and stir well and serve.

Flavorful Turkey and Cranberry Sauce

Servings: 8

Preparation Time: 1 hour

Per Serving: Calories 382, fat 12.6, fiber 9.6, carbs 26.6, protein 17.6

Ingredients:

- 2 Cups chicken stock
- 4 Tablespoons avocado oil
- 1 Cup cranberry sauce
- 2 Big turkey breasts, skinless, boneless and sliced
- 2 Yellow onions, roughly chopped
- Salt and black pepper to the taste

Procedure:

1. Firstly, heat up a pan with the avocado oil over medium-high heat, add the onion and sauté for 5 minutes.
2. Then, add the turkey and brown for 5 minutes more.
3. Now, add the rest of the ingredients, toss, introduce in the oven at 350 degrees F and cook for 40 minutes

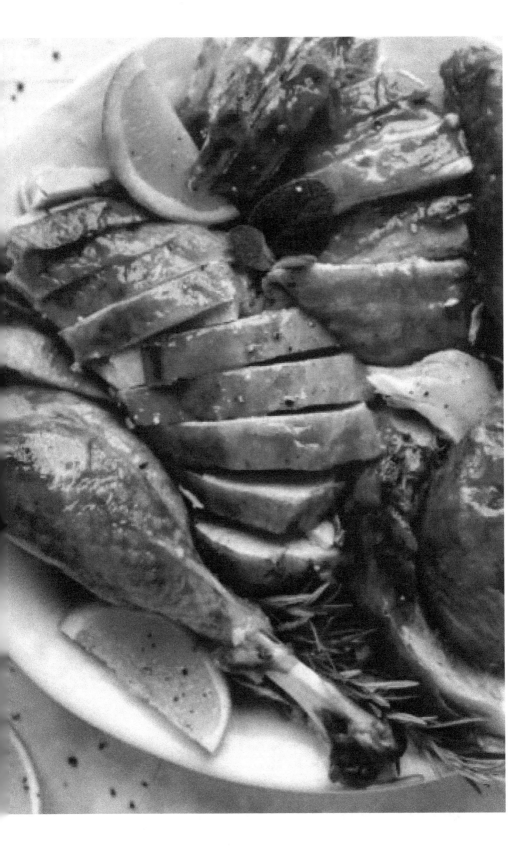

Tasty Sage Turkey Mix

Servings: 8

Preparation Time: 50 minutes

Per Serving: : Calories 382, fat 12.6, fiber 9.6, carbs 16.6, protein 33.2

Ingredients:

- 2 Big turkey breasts, skinless, boneless and roughly cubed
- Juice of 1 lemon
- 4 Tablespoons avocado oil
- 2 Red onions, chopped
- 4 Tablespoons sage, chopped
- 2 Garlic cloves, minced
- 2 Cups chicken stock

Procedure:

1. Firstly, heat up a pan with the avocado oil over medium-high heat, add the turkey and brown for 3 minutes on each side.

2. Then, add the rest of the ingredients, bring to a simmer and cook over medium heat for 35 minutes.
3. Now, divide the mix between plates and serve with a side dish.

Delectable Turkey and Asparagus Mix

Servings: 8

Preparation Time: 40 minutes

Per Serving: : Calories 337, fat 21.2, fiber 10.2, carbs 21.4, protein 17.6

Ingredients:

- 2 Bunch asparagus, trimmed and halved
- 2 Big turkey breasts, skinless, boneless and cut into strips
- 2 Teaspoons basil, dried
- 4 Tablespoons olive oil
- A pinch of salt and black pepper
- 1 Cup tomato sauce
- 2 Tablespoons chives, chopped

Procedure:

1. Firstly, heat up a pan with the oil over medium-high heat, add the turkey and brown for 4 minutes.

2. Then, add the asparagus and the rest of the ingredients except the chives, bring to a simmer and cook over medium heat for 25 minutes.
3. Now, add the chives, divide the mix between plates and serve.

Flavorful Chicken and Mint Sauce

Servings: 8

Preparation Time: 40 minutes

Per Serving: Calories 278, fat 12, fiber 11.2, carbs 18.1, protein 13.3

Ingredients:

- 5 Tablespoons olive oil
- 4 Pounds chicken breasts, skinless, boneless and halved
- 6 Tablespoons garlic, minced
- 4 Tablespoons lemon juice
- 2 Tablespoons red wine vinegar
- 1/3 Cup Greek yogurt
- 4 Tablespoons mint, chopped
- A pinch of salt and black pepper

Procedure:

1. Firstly, in a blender, combine the garlic with the lemon juice and the other ingredients except the oil and the chicken and pulse well.

2. Then, heat up a pan with the oil over medium-high heat, add the chicken and brown for 3 minutes on each side.
3. Add the mint sauce, introduce in the oven and bake everything at 370 degrees F for 25 minutes.
4. Now, divide the mix between plates and serve.

Easy Potato and Kale Bowls

Servings: 8

Preparation Time: 10 minutes

Per Serving: calories: 259 | fat: 5.5g | protein: 7.9g | carbs: 47.6g | fiber: 7.6g | sodium: 1422mg

Ingredients:

- 2 Tablespoons olive oil
- 2 Small onions, peeled and diced
- 2 Stalk celerys, diced
- 4 Cloves garlic, minced
- 8 Medium potatoes, peeled and diced
- 4 Bunches kale, washed, deveined, and chopped
- 3 Cups vegetable broth
- 4 Teaspoons salt
- 1 Teaspoon ground black pepper
- 1/2 Teaspoon caraway seeds
- 2 Tablespoons apple cider vinegar
- 8 Tablespoons sour cream

Procedure:

1. Firstly, dress the Sauté button on Instant Pot.
2. Then, heat oil. Add onion and celery and stir-fry for 3 to 5 minutes until onions are translucent.
3. Add garlic and cook for an additional minute.
4. Add potatoes in an even layer. Add chopped kale in an even layer.
5. Add broth.
6. Lock lid.
7. Press the Manual button and adjust the time to 5 minutes. Let the pressure release naturally for 10 minutes.
8. Quickly release any additional pressure until float valve drops and then unlock lid; then drain broth.
9. Finally, stir in salt, pepper, caraway seeds, and vinegar; slightly mash the potatoes in the Instant Pot.
10. Now, garnish each serving with 1 tablespoon sour cream.

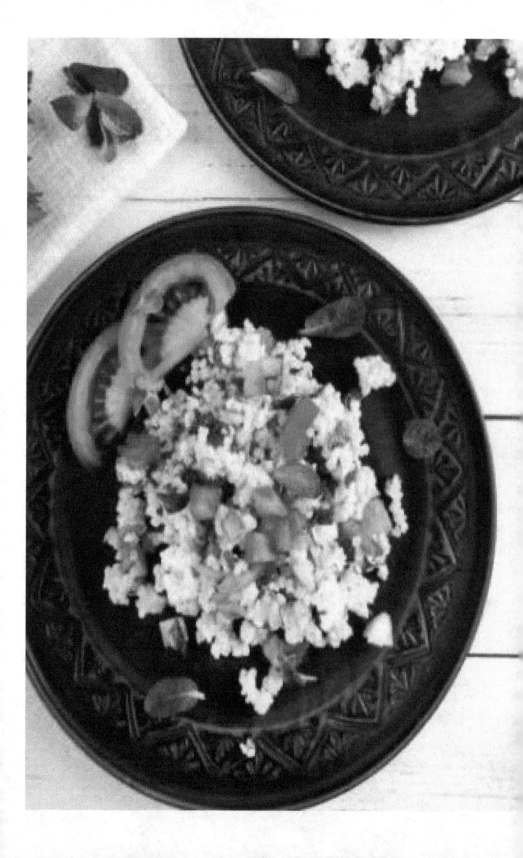

Tasty Eggplant and Millet Pilaf

Servings: 8

Preparation Time: 20 minutes

Per Serving: calories: 238 | fat: 5.6g | protein: 6.0g | carbs: 40.8g | fiber: 5.3g | sodium: 861mg

Ingredients:

- 2 Tablespoons olive oil
- 1/2 Cup peeled and diced onion
- 2 Cups peeled and diced eggplant
- 2 Small Roma tomatoes, seeded and diced
- 2 Cups millet
- 4 Cups vegetable broth
- 2 Teaspoons sea salt
- 1/2 Teaspoon ground black pepper
- 1/4 Teaspoon saffron
- 1/4 Teaspoon cayenne pepper
- 2 Tablespoons chopped fresh chives

Procedure:

1. Firstly, press Sauté button on Instant Pot. Add the olive oil.
2. Then, add onion and cook for 3 to 5 minutes until translucent.
3. Toss in eggplant and stir-fry for 2 more minutes. Add diced tomato.
4. Add millet to Instant Pot in an even layer. Gently pour in broth. Lock lid.
5. Press the Rice button (the Instant Pot will determine the time, about 10 minutes pressurized cooking time).
6. When the timer beeps, let the pressure release naturally for 5 minutes. Quickly release any additional pressure until float valve drops and then unlock lid.
7. Finally, transfer pot ingredients to a serving bowl.
8. Season with salt, pepper, saffron, and cayenne pepper.
9. Now, garnish with chives.

Delicious Grilled Lemon Chicken

Servings: 4

Preparation Time: 20 minutes

Per Serving: calories: 251 | fat: 15.5g | protein: 27.3g | carbs: 1.9g | fiber: 1.0g | sodium: 371mg

Ingredients:

- 4 (4-ounce / 113-g) boneless, skinless chicken breasts
- Marinade:
- 8 Tablespoons freshly squeezed lemon juice
- 24 Tablespoons olive oil, plus more for greasing the grill grates
- 2 Teaspoons dried basil
- 2 Teaspoons paprika
- 1 Teaspoon dried thyme
- 1/2 Teaspoon salt
- ½ Teaspoon garlic powder

Procedure:

1. Firstly, make the marinade: Whisk together the lemon juice, olive oil, basil, paprika, thyme, salt, and garlic powder in a large bowl until well combined.
2. Then, add the chicken breasts to the bowl and let marinate for at least 30 minutes.
3. When ready to cook, preheat the grill to medium-high heat. Lightly grease the grill grates with olive oil.
4. Discard the marinade and arrange the chicken breasts on the grill grates.
5. Finally, grill for 12 to 14 minutes, flipping the chicken halfway through or until a meat thermometer inserted in the center of the chicken reaches 165ºF (74ºC).
6. Now, let the chicken cool for 5 minutes and serve warm.

Tempting Quick Chicken Salad Wraps

Servings: 4

Preparation Time: 15 minutes

Per Serving: calories: 428 | fat: 10.6g | protein: 31.1g | carbs: 50.9g | fiber: 6.0g | sodium: 675mg

Ingredients:

- Tzatziki Sauce:
- 1 Cup plain Greek yogurt
- 2 Tablespoons freshly squeezed lemon juice
- Pinch garlic powder
- 2 Teaspoons dried dill
- Salt and freshly ground black pepper, to taste
- Salad Wraps:
- 4 (8-inch) whole-grain pita bread
- 2 Cups shredded chicken meat
- 4 Cups mixed greens
- 4 Roasted red bell peppers, thinly sliced
- 1 English cucumber, peeled if desired and thinly sliced
- 1/2 Cup pitted black olives
- 2 Scallions, chopped

Procedure:

1. Firstly, make the tzatziki sauce: In a bowl, whisk together the yogurt, lemon juice, garlic powder, dill, salt, and pepper until creamy and smooth.
2. Then, make the salad wraps: Place the pita bread on a clean work surface and spoon ¼ cup of the tzatziki sauce onto each piece of pita bread, spreading it all over.
3. Finally, top with the shredded chicken, mixed greens, red pepper slices, cucumber slices, black olives, finished with chopped scallion.
4. Now, roll the salad wraps and enjoy.

DINNER

Yummy Lemon Marinated Chicken Kebabs

Servings: 8

Preparation Time: 2 hours

Per Serving:

Ingredients:

- 2 Pound chicken breasts, cut into cubes
- 4 Tbsps olive oil
- 4 Cloves garlic, minced
- 1 Cup lemon juice
- Salt and black pepper to taste
- 2 Tsps fresh rosemary, chopped to garnish
- 2 Lemons, cut into wedges to garnish

Procedure:

1. Firstly, thread the chicken onto skewers and set it aside. In a bowl, mix half of the oil, garlic, salt, pepper, and lemon juice, and add the chicken skewers.
2. Then, cover the bowl and let the chicken marinate for at least 2 hours in the refrigerator.

3. When the marinating time is almost over, preheat a grill to 350ºF, and remove the chicken onto the grill. Cook for 6 minutes on each side.
4. Now, remove and serve warm garnished with rosemary leaves and lemons wedges.

Easy Veggie Chicken Drumsticks with Tomato Sauce

Servings: 8

Preparation Time: 1.5 hours

Per Serving:

Ingredients:

- 2 White onions, chopped
- 4 Potatoes, peeled and diced
- 8 Baby carrots, chopped in 1-inch pieces
- 4 Bell peppers, seeded, cut into chunks
- 4 Cloves garlic, minced
- 16 Chicken drumsticks
- 3 Tbsps olive oil
- 1/2 Cup flour
- 2 Cups chicken broth
- 2(28 oz) can tomato sauce
- 4 Tbsps dried Italian herbs
- Salt and black pepper to taste

Procedure:

1. Firstly, heat the oil in a skillet over medium heat, season the drumsticks with salt and pepper, and fry on both sides for 10 minutes.
2. Remove to a baking dish.
3. Then, sauté the onion, potatoes, bell peppers, carrots, and garlic in the same oil and cook for 10 minutes, stirring often.
4. Preheat oven to 400ºF.
5. In a bowl, combine the broth, flour, tomato paste, and Italian herbs together, and pour it over the vegetables in the pan.
6. Stir and cook to thicken for 4 minutes.
7. Finally, pour the mixture on the chicken in the baking dish.
8. Now, bake the chicken and vegetables for around 1 hour.

Delicious Bresaola and Gorgonzola Cake

Servings: 10

Preparation Time: 25 minutes

Per Serving: Calories 240, Fat: 15.3g; Total Carbs: 10g; Protein: 16.1g

Ingredients:

- 4 Tbsps olive oil
- 1 Cup flour
- 6 Slices bresaola, chopped
- 8 Eggs, beaten
- 2 Tsps baking powder
- 2 Cups gorgonzola cheese
- 1/2 Tsp salt
- 1/2 Tsp grated nutmeg

Procedure:

1. Firstly, preheat oven to 390ºF. In a bowl, mix all the ingredients, except for the olive oil.
2. Then, grease cake molds with olive oil, fill them with batter (¾ full) and bake for 15 minutes.
3. Now, let cool completely before serving.

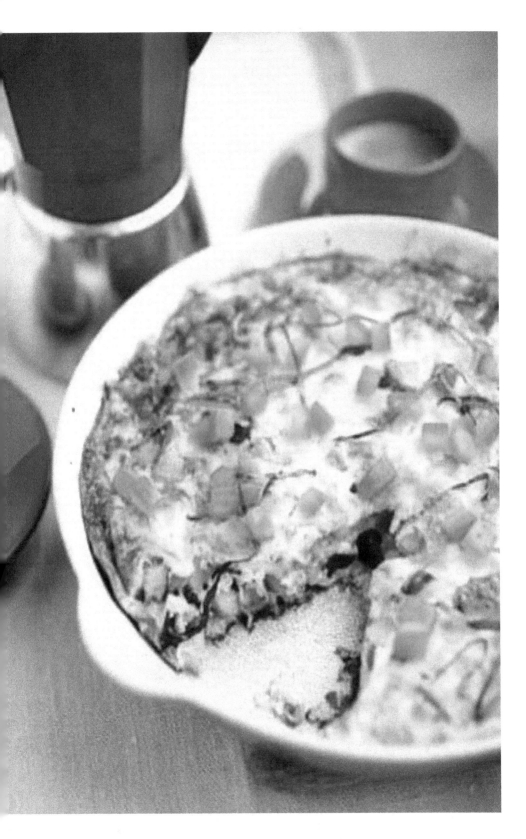

Tempting Spring Frittata

Servings: 4

Preparation Time: 15 minutes

Per Serving: Calories 319; Fat: 25g; Total Carbs: 20g; Protein: 14.9g

Ingredients:

- 4 Tsps olive oil
- 4 Spring onions, chopped
- 4 Spring garlic, chopped
- 8 Eggs, beaten
- 2 Cups yogurt
- 2 Tomatoes, sliced
- 2 Green chili pepper, minced
- 4 Tbsps fresh basil, chopped
- Salt and black pepper, to taste

Procedure:

1. Firstly, let a pan over high heat and warm the olive oil. Sauté garlic and onions until tender.
2. Whisk the eggs with yogurt.

3. Pour into the pan and cook until eggs become puffy and brown to the bottom.
4. Then, add basil, chili pepper and tomatoes to one side of the omelet.
5. Now, add in pepper and salt. Fold the omelet in half and slice into wedges.

Pleasant Blueberry Frittata Flambé

Servings: 6

Preparation Time: 10 minutes

Per Serving: Calories 428, Fat: 32g; Total Carbs: 18g; Protein: 15.3g

Ingredients:

- 12 Eggs, beaten
- 1/2 Cup milk
- 1 Tsp ground cloves
- 2 tbsps olive oil
- 4 tbsps mascarpone cheese
- 36 fresh blueberries
- 2 tbsps powdered sugar
- 2 Tbsps brandy

Procedure:

1. Firstly, set pan over medium heat and warm oil. Mix the eggs with ground cloves and milk.
2. Then, place in the egg mixture; cook for 3 minutes.

3. Set the omelet onto a plate; apply a topping of blueberries and mascarpone cheese. Roll it up and sprinkle with powdered sugar. Pour the warm brandy over the omelet and ignite it.

4. Now, let the flame die out and serve.

Easy Herbs Stuffed Roast Chicken

Servings: 4

Preparation Time: 70 minutes

Per Serving: Calories 432, Fat: 32g; Total Carbs: 15.1g; Protein: 30g

Ingredients:

- 2 Pounds whole chicken
- 1/2 Handful of oregano
- 1/2 Handful of thyme
- 1/2 Handful of parsley
- 1/2 tbsp olive oil
- 1 Pounds cabbage, shredded
- 1/2 Lemon
- 2 Tbsps butter

Procedure:

1. Firstly, stuff the chicken with oregano, thyme, and lemon. Make sure the wings are tucked over and behind.

2. Then, preheat the oven to 450ºF. Roast the chicken for 15 minutes.
3. Reduce the heat to 325ºF and cook for 20 minutes.
4. Spread the butter over the chicken, and sprinkle parsley; add the cabbage.
5. Return to the oven and bake for 30 more minutes.
6. Now, let sit for 10 minutes before carving.

Yummy Halloumi Grape Tomato and Zucchini Skewers

Servings: 8

Preparation Time: 10 minutes

Per Serving: Info:Per Serving:192.2Cal, 20 g total fat (4 g sat. fat), 1 g carb., 1 g fiber, 1 g sugar, 3 g protein, and 328.8 mg sodium.

Ingredients:

- 1/2 Large zucchini, halved lengthways, cut into 8 pieces
- 8 Grape tomatoes
- 90 G halloumi cheese, cut into 16 pieces
- Olive oil spray
- For the spinach-basil oil:
- 1 Cup baby spinach leaves
- 1 Cup fresh basil leaves
- 185 ml (3/4 cup) extra-virgin olive oil
- 125 ml (1/2 cup) light olive oil

Procedure:

1. Firstly, in a saucepan of boiling water, cook the spinach and the basil for about 30 seconds or until just wilted.
2. Then, drain and cool under running cold water.
3. Place the cooked spinach and basil into a food processor.
4. Add the light olive oil and the extra-virgin olive oil; process until the mixture is smooth.
5. Finally, transfer into an airtight container, refrigerate for 8 hours to develop the flavors.
6. Preheat the barbecue grill to medium-high.
7. Thread a piece of zucchini, halloumi cheese, and tomato into each skewer. Lightly spray with the olive oil spray.
8. Grill for about4 minutes per side or until cooked through and golden brown.
9. Now, arrange the grilled skewers on to serving platter; serve immediately with the prepared spinach-basil oil.

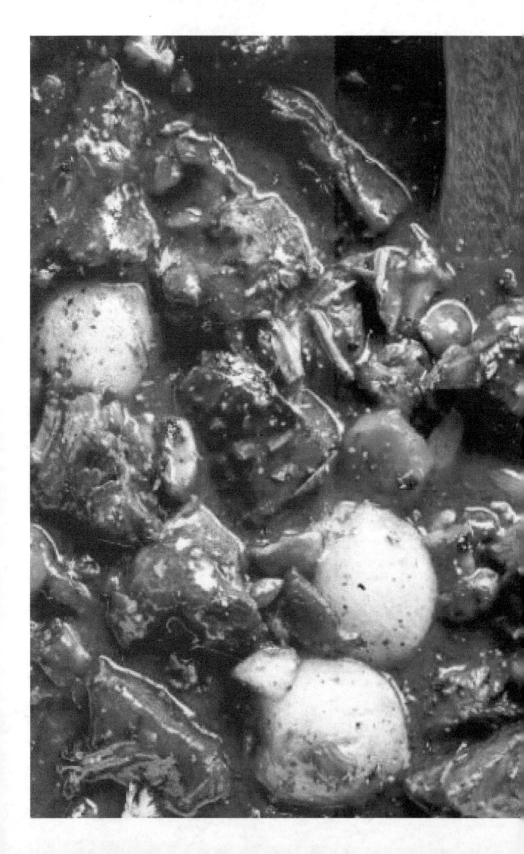

Beef Bourguignon

Servings: 8

Preparation Time: 2 hours

Per Serving: Calories:306   Fat:12.6g   Protein:37.6g   Carbohydrates:9.0g

Ingredients:

- 3 sweet onions, chopped
- 2 carrots, sliced
- 4 garlic cloves, minced
- 1 chili pepper, sliced
- 1 pound button mushrooms
- 1 ½ cups beef stock
- ½ cup dark beer
- 2 bay leaves
- 1 thyme sprig
- 1 rosemary sprig
- Salt and pepper to taste
- 3 tablespoons olive oil
- 2 pounds beef roast, cubed
- 1 tablespoon all-purpose flour

Procedure:

1. Sprinkle the beef with flour.
2. Heat the oil in a deep heavy pot and add the beef roast.
3. Cook on all sides for 5 minutes or until browned.
4. Add the onions, carrots and chili and cook for 5 more minutes.
5. Add the mushrooms, stock, beer, bay leaves, thyme, rosemary, salt and pepper.
6. Cover the pot and cook on low heat for 1 ½ hours.
7. Serve the stew warm and fresh.

Flank Steak

Servings: 4

Preparation Time: 40 minutes

Per Serving: Calories:234   Fat:13.4g   Protein:21.6g
Carbohydrates:6.7g

Ingredients:

- 1 teaspoon Dijon mustard
- 1 teaspoon chopped thyme
- 1 teaspoon dried sage
- 4 garlic cloves, chopped
- 2 tablespoons olive oil
- Salt and pepper to taste
- 4 flank steaks
- 1 lemon, juiced
- 1 orange, juiced

Procedure:

1. First, combine the flank steaks and the rest of the ingredients in a zip lock bag.
2. Then refrigerate for 30 minutes.

3. Now heat a grill pan over medium flame and place the steaks on the grill.
4. Cook on each side for 6-7 minutes.
5. Serve the steaks warm and fresh.

Grilled Salmon with Cucumber Dill Sauce

Servings: 4

Preparation Time: 40 minutes

Per   Serving: Calories:224   Fat:10.3g   Protein:26.3g
Carbohydrates:8.9g

Ingredients:

- ½ cup Greek yogurt
- 1 tablespoon lemon juice
- 1 tablespoon olive oil
- 4 salmon fillets
- 1 teaspoon smoked paprika
- 1 teaspoon dried sage
- Salt and pepper to taste
- 4 cucumbers, sliced
- 2 tablespoons chopped dill

Procedure:

1. First, season the salmon with salt, pepper, paprika and sage.

2. Then heat a grill pan over medium flame and place the salmon on the grill.

3. Now cook on each side for 4 minutes.

4. For the sauce, mix the cucumbers, dill, yogurt, lemon juice and oil in a bowl. Add salt and pepper and mix well.

5. Serve the salmon with the cucumber sauce.

Basil-Lemon Grilled Tofu Burger

Servings: 6

Preparation Time: 6 minutes

Per Serving: 276 Cal, 11.3 g total fat (1.9 g sat. fat, 5.7 g mono fat, 2.2 g poly fat), 10.5 g protein, 34.5 g carb., 1.5 g fiber, 5 mg chol., 2.4 mg iron, 743 mg sodium, and 101 mg calcium.

Ingredients:

- 1/3 cup fresh basil, finely chopped
- 2 tablespoons Dijon mustard
- 2 tablespoons honey
- 1/4 cup freshly squeezed lemon juice
- 1 garlic cloves, minced
- 1/3 cup Kalamata olives, finely, chopped pitted
- 1 cup watercress, trimmed
- Cooking spray
- 2 teaspoons grated lemon rind
- 1 tablespoon olive oil, extra-virgin,
- 1/2 teaspoon salt
- 1/4 teaspoon black pepper (freshly ground)
- 3 garlic cloves, minced

- 3 tablespoons sour cream, reduced-fat
- 3 tablespoons light mayonnaise
- 6 slices (1/4-inch thick each) tomato
- 6 pieces (1 1/2-ounce) whole-wheat hamburger buns
- 1 pound tofu, firm or extra-firm, drained

Procedure:

1. Combine the marinade ingredients in a small-sized bowl. In a crosswise direction, cut the tofu into 6 slices.
2. Pat each piece dry using paper towels.
3. Place them in a jelly roll pan and brush both sides of the slices with the marinade mixture; reserve any leftover marinade.
4. Marinate for 1 hour.
5. Preheat the grill and coated the grill rack with cooking spray.
6. Place the tofu slices; grill for about 3 minutes per side, brushing the tofu with the reserved marinade mixture.
7. In a small-sized bowl, combine the garlic-olive mayonnaise ingredients.
8. Spread about 1 1/2 tablespoons of the mixture over the bottom half of the hamburger buns.
9. Top each with 1 slice tofu, 1 slice tomato, about 2 tablespoons of watercress, and top with the top buns.

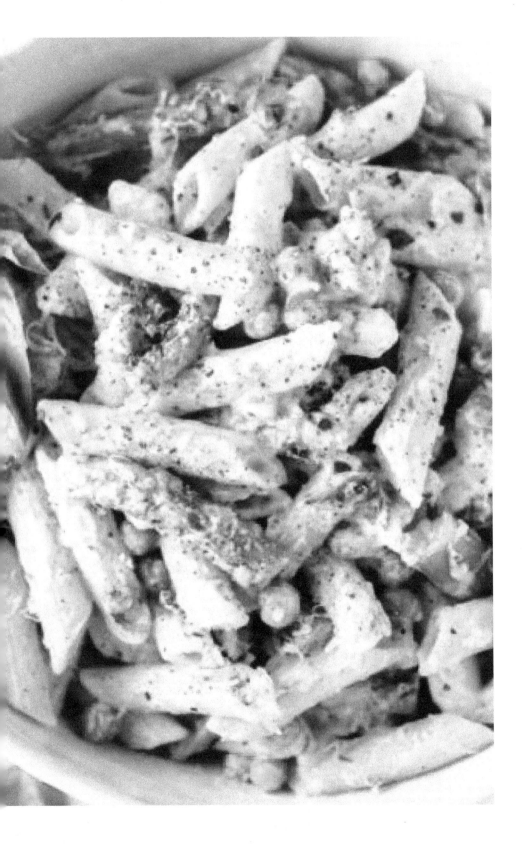

Green Pea Creamy Pasta

Servings: 4

Preparation Time: 25 minutes

Per Serving: Calories:294 Fat:20.1g Protein:6.4g
Carbohydrates:25.9g

Ingredients:

- 2 tablespoons olive oil
- 2 garlic cloves, chopped
- 2 mint leaves
- 1 tablespoon lemon juice
- 2 tablespoons vegetable stock
- Salt and pepper to taste
- 8 oz. whole wheat spaghetti
- 1 cup green peas
- 1 avocado, peeled and cubed
- ¼ cup heavy cream

Procedure:

1. First, pour a few cups of water in a deep pot and bring to a boil with a pinch of salt.

2. Then add the spaghetti and cook for 8 minutes, then drain well.
3. Now for the sauce, combine the remaining ingredients in a blender and pulse until smooth.
4. Mix the cooked spaghetti with the sauce and serve the pasta fresh.

CPSIA information can be obtained
at www.ICGtesting.com
Printed in the USA
BVHW012056230521
607866BV00030B/1207